MRCP Cardiolog...

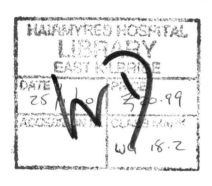

MRCP Cardiology MCQs

STEPHEN BRENNAN

MBChB, BSc(Pharm), MPSI, MRPharmS,
Cert Med Ed, MRCS(Ed)

Specialist Registrar in General Surgery
Aberdeen Royal Infirmary

Radcliffe Publishing
Oxford • New York

Radcliffe Publishing Ltd
18 Marcham Road
Abingdon
Oxon OX14 1AA
United Kingdom

www.radcliffe-oxford.com

Electronic catalogue and worldwide online ordering facility.

British Library Cataloguing in Publication Data

A catalogue record for this book is available from the British Library.

ISBN-13: 978 184619 358 3

The paper used for the text pages of this book is FSC certified. FSC (The Forest Stewardship Council) is an international network to promote responsible management of the world's forests.

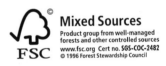

Mixed Sources
Product group from well-managed forests and other controlled sources
www.fsc.org Cert no. SGS-COC-2482
© 1996 Forest Stewardship Council

Typeset by Pindar NZ, Auckland, New Zealand
Printed and bound by TJI Digital, Padstow, Cornwall, UK

Contents

Preface

MRCP Cardiology MCQs is written as a study aid specifically for candidates studying for Membership examinations of the Royal Colleges. It contains 150 multiple choice questions (MCQs), each with various numbers of stem answers. Cardiology is a large and critical branch of internal medicine and covers such a vast amount of knowledge that I believe it warrants a book to itself, although an equal depth of knowledge is required in other areas in order to pass.

The questions are designed to cover a wide range of both cardiology and cardiovascular pharmacology and encompass both basic anatomy and physiology of the heart, through to advanced topics such as evidence-based medicine. The questions are supplemented at the back of the book with explanatory answers to aid further revision and study.

Good luck with the exams!

Stephen Brennan
June 2009

About the author

Stephen Brennan initially graduated in Pharmacology and then studied Medicine at the University of Aberdeen. After training in cardiothoracic surgery, he is currently a Specialist Registrar in General Surgery with a particular interest in colorectal surgery and the general surgery of childhood. In addition, he is involved with both undergraduate and postgraduate surgical training and is a tutor for the Royal College of Surgeons of Edinburgh and MRCS revision courses. He is an instructor in Advanced Trauma Life Support (ATLS) and has completed a postgraduate qualification in medical education.

Acknowledgement

The author would like to greatly acknowledge and thank consultant cardiologist Dr Kevin Jennings for his help in proofreading the original manuscript.

Dedicated to Derv and Joe

SECTION 1

Cardiovascular pharmacology

Cardiac glycosides

Q1 Digoxin:

    a Shortens the PR interval

    b Should be stopped prior to elective DC cardioversion

    c May cause atrial fibrillation

    d May cause false-positive results on exercise testing

    e Can only be administered orally

Q2 Digoxin toxicity:

    a May cause ventricular fibrillation

    b May cause ventricular tachycardia

    c May cause atrial fibrillation

    d May be precipitated by hypokalaemia

    e May be precipitated by hypercalcaemia

Q3 Digoxin:

    a Acts by inhibiting the enzyme H/K-ATPase

    b Has a positive chronotropic effect

    c Has a negative inotropic effect

    d In high doses, increases the sympathetic outflow from the central nervous system

    e Peak serum concentrations occur in 20–30 minutes

Q4 Digoxin:

   a Reduces mortality in cardiac failure

   b May be used as a second-line agent in WPW syndrome

   c Withdrawal of digoxin from patients with chronic heart failure may be associated with cardiac decompensation

   d Toxicity treated with Digibind may result in hyperkalaemia

   e Toxicity does not occur if the plasma concentration levels are in the correct therapeutic range

Q5 Digoxin toxicity may be precipitated by:

   a A creatinine level of 180 mmol/L

   b A potassium level of 6.2 mmol/L

   c Co-administration of verapamil

   d Co-administration of warfarin

   e Acute lobar pneumonia

Q6 Which of the following occur following regular digoxin medication?

   a Increased force and rate of contraction

   b Decreased heart rate

   c Increased automaticity

   d a and b

   e All of the above

Q7 Digoxin causes which of the following ECG changes?

a   T-wave flattening

b   Prolonged PR interval

c   Shortened QT interval

d   Tenting of the T-wave

Q8 Digoxin causes which of the following physiological effects?

a   Decreasing aldosterone levels

b   Direct renal vasodilation

c   Inhibiting ADH levels

d   Increasing cardiac output

Diuretics

Q9 Frusemide:

    a Is a short-acting thiazide diuretic

    b Typically causes hypercalcaemia

    c May precipitate digoxin toxicity

    d Acts on the descending limb of the Loop of Henle

    e May cause glucose intolerance

Q10 Thiazide diuretics cause the following electrolyte disturbances:

    a Hypoglycaemia

    b Hyponatraemia

    c Hypokalaemia

    d Hypocalcaemia

    e Hypouricaemia

Q11 The cardiotoxic effects of digoxin are enhanced in the presence of:

    a Hyperkalaemia

    b Hypercalcaemia

    c Alkalosis

    d Hypokalaemia

    e Hyperchloraemia

Q12 Metolazone:

    a Is only active by the IV route

    b Is an orally active loop diuretic

    c Acts synergistically with frusemide

    d Is contraindicated in renal failure

    e Is licenced for acute pulmonary oedema

Q13 Bendrofluazide:

    a Is initially started at 5 mg daily in the management of hypertension

    b Is a long-acting loop diuretic

    c Tends to cause hyponatraemia, hypocalcaemia, and hyperuricaemia

    d Male impotence is a *rare* side effect

    e May be given as an IV bolus in acute pulmonary oedema

Q14 Spironolactone:

    a Is a long-acting thiazide diuretic

    b May cause hyperkalaemia

    c Is a first-line agent for essential hypertension

    d Is used in the treatment of Conn's syndrome

    e Has no role in the management of ascites secondary to alcoholic cirrhosis

Beta-adrenoceptor blocking drugs

Q15 Propranolol is contraindicated in the presence of:

a   Complete heart block

b   Peripheral vascular disease

c   Diabetes mellitus

d   Atrial fibrillation

e   Asthma

Q16 Cardioselective beta-blockers are contraindicated in:

a   Asthma

b   Diabetes mellitus

c   Male erectile impotence

d   Peripheral vascular disease

e   Migraines

Q17 The rationale for giving atenolol with nicardipine in treating hypertension is to:

a   Cause peripheral vasoconstriction

b   Decrease renin release

c   Prevent reflex tachycardia

d   Decrease mortality

e   Decrease side-effect profile

Q18 The following beta-blockers are associated with a proven significant mortality reduction post-MI:

a Atenolol

b Propranolol

c Timolol

d Carvedilol

e Metoprolol

Q19 Propranolol:

a Crosses the blood–brain barrier more readily than atenolol

b Is long acting and may be given once daily for the treatment of hypertension

c May cause hypothyroidism

d Is a first-line agent in the treatment of benign familial tremor

e Is a recognised cause of psoriasis

Q20 Beta-blockers post-MI showed the following results:

a The MIAMI trial showed significant mortality reduction with metoprolol post-MI

b The Gotenburg metoprolol trial showed that metoprolol conferred a significantly lower rate of ventricular fibrillation arrest post-MI

c The GREAT trial demonstrated a significant mortality reduction using oral timolol post non-q wave MI

d ISIS-1 demonstrated benefits with early use of atenolol post-MI

e Beta-blockers must be avoided in post-MI patients where the ejection fraction is less than 40%

Q21 Carvedilol:

a Is a non-selective beta- and alpha-adrenoceptor antagonist

b Has no intrinsic sympathomimetic activity

c Exerts calcium-channel blocking activity at high dosages

d Is highly protein bound

e Has no antioxidant properties

Calcium-channel antagonists

Q22 Verapamil:

a Commonly causes diarrhoea as a side effect

b Has weak negative inotropic properties

c Increases the renal excretion of digoxin by up to 100%

d Is an effective treatment of WPW syndrome

e Is an effective treatment for SVT

Q23 Common side effects of calcium-channel blockers include:

a Flushing

b Anaphylaxis

c Oedema

d Diarrhoea

e Headache

Q24 Diltiazem:

a Has a greater negative inotropic effect than verapamil

b Is a class III antidysrhythmic agent

c Has a greater negative inotropic effect than nifedipine

d Reduces mortality post non-Q wave MI

e May be given by slow IV injection for the rapid cardioversion of SVT

Q25 Amlodipine:

a Is the longest-acting calcium-channel blocker in UK clinical practice

b Has a half-life of 24 hours

c Has a starting dose for hypertension of 100 mg daily (50 mg daily in renal impairment)

d Is contraindicated in dilated cardiomyopathy

e Is safe for patients with severe CCF

Q26 The following statements about verapamil are correct:

a It is not effective when administered IV

b It causes decreased AV-nodal conduction

c It is contraindicated in asthma

d It may cause bradycardia

e It is primarily metabolised by the kidneys

Q27 Nicorandil:

a Is a potassium-channel activator that contains a nitrate as part of its molecular structure

b Causes headache as its most common side effect

c Has a half-life of 24 hours

d Reduces all-cause mortality post-PTCA

e May cause hypothroidism

Q28 A 55-year-old man is on multiple drug therapy. Which of the following is most likely to induce microsomal enzymes?

a Allopurinol

b Cimetidine

c Clarithromycin

d Ketoconazole

e Phenytoin

ACE inhibitors

Q29 ACE inhibitors have clinically significant interactions with:

a Diclofenac

b Digoxin

c Lithium

d Erythromycin

e Carbimazole

Q30 ACE inhibitors:

a Cause cough in about 10% of patients

b Cause hypokalaemia in about 1% of patients

c Are safe for patients with asthma

d Cause diarrhoea as the most common side effect

e Cause headache as the most common side effect

Q31 The TRACE study:

a Used lisinopril as its ACE inhibitor

b Had confirmed MI in all patients

c Had echo confirmed decreased ejection fraction in all patients

d Examined low-risk post-MI patients

e Included patients with a mean age of 55 years

Q32 The SMILE study:

a Compared zofenopril with placebo in patients with acute anterior MI

b Used MI patients who were not suitable for thrombolysis

c Excluded patients presenting greater than 6 hours after onset of symptoms

d Showed that zofenopril reduced 24-hour mortality by 83% post acute MI

e Showed that the incidence of cough was 12% in the zofenopril group

Q33 What effects does quinapril have on serum renin and angiotensin II, respectively?

a Decrease; decrease

b Increase; increase

c Increase; decrease

d Decrease; increase

e Decrease; no change

Q34 Regarding the HOPE trial:

a All patients had MI or stroke within the previous 4 weeks

b This study also tested the effect of vitamin E supplementation

c Overall mortality was reduced by about 20%

d Incidence of CHF was lower in the ramipril group

e Complications of diabetes, including nephropathy, retinopathy requiring laser, and dialysis, were all lower in the ramipril group

Statins

Q35 Simvastatin:

a Is derived synthetically from the fermentation product of *Aspergillus terreus*

b Is a specific inhibitor of HMG-CoA reductase, the enzyme that catalyzes the conversion of HMG-CoA to melandronic acid

c Has a cholesterol-lowering effect usually seen within 2 weeks, with maximum therapeutic response occurring within 6 months

d Should be continued during pregnancy in a patient with primary hypercholesterolaemia

e May cause fatal rhabdomyolysis in about 1 in 10 000 patients

Q36 Atorvastatin:

a Produced greater reductions in total cholesterol than fluvastatin, pravastatin, or simvastatin in large, comparative trials

b Results in about 90% of the maximum observed reductions in LDL being attained within the first 2 weeks of therapy

c Is >98% bound to plasma proteins and is extensively metabolised by cytochrome P450 3A4 to active metabolites

d Is available as white, film-coated 10, 20 and 40 mg tablets

Q37 The CARE study:

a Was a randomised, double-blind, placebo-controlled primary prevention trial of lowering normal plasma cholesterol levels following MI

b Used atorvastatin as its active agent

c   Showed that the frequency of fatal coronary events was reduced by 50% in the active drug-treated group

d   Showed that the frequency of CABG was reduced by 26%

e   Showed that the frequency of PTCA was reduced by 23%

Q38 The 4S Trial:

a   Is a primary prevention study involving 4444 patients

b   Evaluated pravastatin versus placebo post-MI

c   Examined patients with cholesterol levels of 5.5–8.0 mmol/L

d   Showed a 37% reduction in the need to undergo re-vascularisation procedures

e   Showed that 1% of patients developed rhabdomyolysis

Q39 The LIPID study:

a   Compared pravastatin 40 mg vs placebo

b   Demonstrated a 12% decrease in hospitalization for unstable angina

c   Examined patients post-MI with high cholesterol levels (>7 mmol/L)

d   Had no effect on overall all-cause mortality

e   Showed that all patients had confirmed MI by WHO criteria

Thrombolytics

Q40 A 75-year-old man with COPD is admitted to A&E Resus with VT complicated by runs of SVT. The drug of choice would be:

a   Adenosine

b   Amiodarone

c   Esmolol

d   Quinidine

e   Adrenaline

Q41 The following are contraindications to thrombolysis:

a   Recent CVA (in the last 6 months)

b   Recent upper GI bleed

c   Prolonged CPR

d   Diabetic retinopathy

e   Ulcerative colitis

Q42 Accelerated rTPA should be used as a first-line agent if:

a   The previous MI thrombolysed with streptokinase 6 months ago

b   There was recent streptococcal infection

c   There was a large inferior infarction presenting within 4 hours

d   Hypotension (SBP <100 mgHg) is present

e   There is a likely need for temporary pacing

Q43 Complications of streptokinase include:

a   Henoch–Schonlein purpura

b   Bronchospasm

c Systemic embolism

d VF arrest

e Pulseless electrical activity

Q44 The GREAT trial:

a Was a randomised, double-blind trial using streptokinase for acute MI

b Showed that the benefit of thrombolytic therapy was most marked when treatment was administered within 2 hours of the onset of symptoms

c Showed that, 1 year after trial entry, 10.4% of patients given anistreplase at home died compared with 21.6% of those given anistreplase in hospital

d Showed that all patients thrombolysed also received heparin 5000 iu IV stat

e Showed that patients receiving a thrombolytic at home received a placebo in hospital

Q45 Heparin-induced thrombocytopenia (HIT):

a May result in life-threatening thrombosis

b Usually occurs after long-term (>3 months) subcutaneous heparin therapy

c May be less likely to occur with low-molecular weight heparin than unfractionated heparin

d May be preceded by thrombosis

e Can be caused by an IgM antibody (immune-mediated HIT)

Anti-platelet agents

Q46 Aspirin:

a Is an irreversible cyclo-oxygenase inhibitor

b Should not be administered simultaneously with warfarin

c Is a reversible phosphodiesterase inhibitor

d Has little or no anti-platelet effect below 75 mg per day

e Is given as 300 mg stat for its rapid sublingual analgesic action post-MI

Q47 Tirofiban (Aggrastat):

a Should not be used in patients with a history of stroke or those who have had a major surgical procedure within the past 30 days

b Is superior to abciximab for patients undergoing PTCA

c Causes more bleeding complications than abciximab

d Is the drug of choice for primary PTCA when used for acute MI

e Reduced all-cause mortality compared to heparin alone for PTCA in the TARGET study

Q48 Eptifibatide:

a Is a cyclic heptapeptide GP IIb/IIIa inhibitor

b Resulted in a 31% reduction in the combined end point of nonfatal MI or death at 30 days in patients undergoing PTCA

c Treatment, when discontinued, causes no further effects either beneficial or detrimental

d   Causes more non-fatal blood dyscrasias than either heparin
    or tirofiban

e   Is a chimeric Fab fragment of a monoclonal antibody to the
    GP IIb/IIIa receptor

Inotropes

Q49 Dopamine:

  a At 10 mcg/kg/min, is maximum dose

  b Has no effect on alpha receptors

  c Must be given into a large peripheral line

  d May be safely used in patients concurrently on MAOIs

  e Has a more potent positive chronotropic effect than noradrenaline

Q50 Isoprenaline:

  a Causes tachycardia

  b Causes hyperglycaemia

  c Is useful for the treatment of bradycardia that is not responsive to atropine

  d Is a B-adrenergic receptor agonist that has a positive inotropic effect, decreases peripheral vascular resistance, and causes pulmonary vasodilation

  e Is incompatible with aminophylline, and sodium bicarbonate

Q51 Atropine:

  a Is a naturally occurring alkaloid of 'atropa belladonna'

  b Is a competitive antagonist of muscarinic cholinergic receptors

  c Is generally effective in adults at a dose level of 250–500 mcg when used to treat bradycardias

  d May result in paradoxical bradycardia at slow IV administration levels and is not recommended

  e May cause flushed dry skin, tachycardia, respiratory depression, blurred vision, constricted pupils, and dry mouth

Q52 Methoxamine:

a Acts on a1 receptors

b May cause a reflex decrease in heart rate, and therefore it is good for hypotension with tachycardia

c Is metabolised by monoamine oxidase

d Is metabolised by cathol-O-methyl transferase

e Is useful in the management of paroxysmal atrial tachycardia

Q53 Regarding dopamine:

a Sodium bicarbonate inactivates dopamine

b MAOIs potentiate the dopamine effect

c Bretylium effects may be synergistic with dopamine

d Dopamine decreases pulmonary artery wedge pressure

e At high doses (10–20 mcg/kg/hr), dopamine causes vasoconstriction of renal and splanchnic beds

Q54 Adenosine:

a Has a half-life of 30 minutes

b Should be avoided in patients with asthma

c Is active orally

d Must be given by slow IV infusion through a large peripheral vein

e Is chemically similar to adrenaline

Q55 Noradrenaline:

    a Is a pure alpha receptor stimulant

    b Is a potent bronchodilator

    c Increases myocardial oxygen consumption

    d Increases skeletal muscle blood flow

    e Increases pulmonary capillary wedge pressure

Q56 Lignocaine:

    a Acts by inhibiting fast sodium channels

    b Prolongs the cardiac action potential

    c Acts more effectively if hypokalaemia is avoided

    d Has a greater negative inotropic effect than disopyramide

    e Acts preferentially on ischaemic myocardium

Anti-dysrythmic drugs

Q57 Signs of quinidine toxicity are:

a Ventricular fibrillation

b Ventricular tachycardia

c Hypotension

d Blurred vision

e Atrial fibrillation

Q58 Bretylium:

a Is a second-line agent for VT arrest resistant to IV lignocaine

b Is available orally for the long-term management of AF

c Has a half-life of 10 minutes

d Has a suitable dose of 300 mg IV bolus for a standard 70 kg adult

e Has hypotension as its most common side effect

Q59 Quinidine is usually contraindicated in:

a Ventricular fibrillation

b Thrombocytopenia

c Concurrent digoxin therapy

Q60 Quinidine:

    a Is a dextrostereoisomer of quinine

    b Is a vinca alkaloid

    c Has muscarinic antagonist properties

    d Is only effective IV

    e Causes a prolonged cardiac refractory period

Q61 Flecainide:

    a Is a fluorinated derivative of procainamide

    b Can reduce mortality if used post-MI to treat pre-mature ventricular ectopic beats

    c Is a class Ib antidysrhythmic agent

    d Terminates AF in up to 50% of patients with WPW syndrome and reduces the ventricular rate in the remainder

    e Is very effective in the treatment of atrial flutter

Q62 Tinnitus is a common side effect of:

    a Digoxin

    b Amiodarone

    c Atenolol

    d Aspirin

    e Quinidine

Q63 Lignocaine is effective in the treatment of:

    a Paroxysmal atrial tachycardia

    b Ventricular tachycardia

    c Premature ventricular beats

d Torsades de pointes

e Atrial flutter

Q64 Disopramide:

a Is a myocardial depressant

b Has anticholinergic side effects

c Toxicity may cause QT-segment prolongation

d Toxicity may occur in the presence of hypokalaemia

e May cause increased bronchial secretions

Q65 Amiodarone has which of the following properties?

a It increases the INR of patients on warfarin

b It enhances the effect of digoxin

c It is composed of iodine

d It causes prolongation of the plateau phase of the cardiac action potential

e It may cause pulmonary fibrosis

Q66 GTN:

a Causes less headache than amyl-nitrate

b Typically causes tolerance after about 6 weeks

c Is synonymous with nitroglycerine

d May cause methaemaglobinaemia

e Is a direct-acting vasodilator

SECTION 2

Cardiology

Acute myocardial infarction

Q67 Acute myocardial infarction:

   a Has a 50% pre-hospital admission mortality

   b Has an in-hospital mortality of 1–5%

   c May be completely asymptomatic

   d May present as an occipital headache

   e May present as a toothache

Q68 Conditions that may mimic symptoms of an MI are:

   a Ruptured oesophagus

   b Perforated duodenal ulcer

   c Gastro-oesophageal reflux disorder

   d Pulmonary embolism

   e Panic attack

Q69 In the management of acute MI:

   a Compared to placebo, aspirin decreases mortality by 50%

   b Early resolution of ST-segment deviation is a greater predictor of mortality than maximum ST elevation at 90 minutes after thrombolysis

   c ST elevation in II, III, AVF has poorer prognosis than anterior infarcts

   d Heart block is more common with anterior wall infarction

   e Presence of ventricular ectopics has no effect on overall prognosis

Q70 Primary PTCA angioplasty in acute MI is preferred if the delay to thrombolysis is less than:

a 30 minutes

b 60 minutes

c 90 minutes

d 120 minutes

e 180 minutes

Q71 In the ISIS-4 trial:

a Oral captopril was started 48 hours after thrombolysis

b Early use of intravenous nitrates showed benefit in patients who presented within 4 hours of the onset of chest pain

c Intravenous magnesium was ineffective

d Captopril started early in acute MI saved about 5 lives per 1000 treated for 1 month

e Was a large study involving 5800 patients demonstrating no benefit from using oral mononitrate

Q72 Hibernating myocardium:

a Is synonymous with myocardial stunning

b Is reversible

c Is rare, occurring in about 1–2% patients with symptomatic ischaemic heart disease

d Is rare after MI

e May be diagnosed using echocardiography

Q73 ST-segment elevation typically occurs in the following conditions:

a   Acute pericarditis

b   Left ventricular hypertrophy

c   Digoxin toxicity

d   Non-Q wave MI

e   Right ventricular hypertrophy

Q74 An acute MI:

a   Can cause chest pain not relieved by GTN

b   May be without chest pain in diabetics

c   Should prompt administration of IM morphine

d   May be diagnosed from the history alone

e   Typically shows on the ECG in the form of Q-waves

Hypertension

Q75 Hypertension:

 a In 95% of cases, no cause can be found

 b Caucasians have a lower BP than a black population living in the same environment

 c Is always asymptomatic

 d Affects 5% of the population

 e May indicate possible Conn's syndrome when associated with hyperkalaemia

Q76 Which of the following would be first-line agents for the management of moderate hypertension?

 a Nifedipine

 b Minoxidil

 c Clonidine

 d Methyldopa

 e Bendrofluazide

Q77 Untreated hypertension may result in:

 a Ruptured aortic aneurysms

 b Renal artery stenosis

 c Conn's syndrome

 d Aortic dissection

Q78 Recognised causes of hypertension include:

 a Excess salt ingestion

 b Oral contraceptive pill

c Alcohol

d Liquorice ingestion

e Smoking

Q79 Regarding hypertension:

a Systolic blood pressure increases throughout life

b Diastolic blood pressure increases to age 50 years, then stabilises

c Newly emergent hypertension after age 65 years is usually isolated systolic hypertension

d There is no mortality reduction to be gained from treating isolated systolic hypertension in the elderly

e There is no mortality benefit to be gained from treating hypertension in patients over 80 years old

Q80 A 60-year-old female with type II diabetes is being treated for hypertension and the prevention of proteinuria associated with diabetic nephropathy. The likely drug is:

a Bendrofluazide

b Ramipril

c Methyldopa

d Atenolol

e Valsartan

Q81 In acromegaly:

    a Diabetes mellitus occurs in about 50% of cases

    b Hypertension occurs in about 30% of cases

    c There is decreased sensitivity to angiotensin II

    d Hypertrophic cardiomyopathy independent of hypertension develops

    e LVH is present in more than half of cases

Q82 Which of the following antihypertensive agents is ideal for the management of a 60-year-old male type II diabetic who has a history of asthma, gout, and hypercholesterolaemia?

    a Atenolol

    b Bendrofluazide

    c Carvedilol

    d Ramipril

    e Verapamil

Q83 A 60-year-old Nigerian is being treated with a drug for essential hypertension. His GP checks routine biochemistry, which shows low serum potassium and high levels of calcium, uric acid, and glucose. The likely agent is:

    a Methyldopa

    b Bumetanide

    c Frusemide

    d Spironolactone

    e Enalapril

Q84 A 60-year-old female has recently been started on an antihypertensive. A few weeks later, she develops joint pains in her arms and legs. Which of the following is the likely cause?

a Ramipril

b Bendrofluazide

c Clonidine

d Nicardipine

e Methyldopa

Atrial fibrillation

Q85 Regarding atrial fibrillation (AF):

   a AF usually complicates acute MI in about 1% of cases

   b Hypertension accounted for about half of the cases of AF in the Framingham study

   c Is typically asymptomatic

   d Resolution to sinus rhythm is less likely if due to thyrotoxicosis rather than to ischaemic heart disease

   e AF is present in 0.4% of adults

Q86 Recognised causes of AF include:

   a Thyrotoxicosis

   b Rheumatic heart disease

   c Alcohol

   d WPW syndrome

   e Atrial myxoma

Q87 Amiodarone:

   a May cause hypothyroidism

   b May cause hyperthyroidism

   c Contains iodine as part of its molecular structure

   d Is strongly negatively inotropic

   e Is a class III antidysrythmic agent

Q88 Recognised side effects of amiodarone are:

   a Pulmonary embolism

   b Pulmonary fibrosis

c Pulmonary atelectasis

d Corneal micro-deposits

e Red man syndrome

Q89 Concerning stroke prevention:

a Aspirin is a cyclo-oxygenase inhibitor, and dipyridamole is a cyclic nucleotide phosphodiesterase inhibitor; when combined, the two agents seem to offer a greater pharmacologic advantage than does either taken alone

b Aspirin with dipyridamole cut patients' risk of stroke and death by one-third, compared with patients taking aspirin plus placebo

c For TIA patients with atrial fibrillation, a target INR of 3.5 is recommended

d Good surgical candidates for carotid endarterectomy have stenosis of 70–99%

e Carotid endarterectomy is suitable for acute management of TIA with 50% stenosis of the ipsilateral common carotid artery

Dysrhythmias

Q90 WPW syndrome:

    a The Kent accessory pathway was first discovered in 1893

    b Occurs in about 1% of the population

    c Type A has the accessory pathway on the left side of the heart

    d Type B has a positive delta wave in lead I

    e May mimic LBBB on the ECG

Q91 First-degree AV block:

    a The AV nodal artery is usually a branch of the right coronary artery

    b Is more common after inferior than anterior MI

    c Is always pathological

    d Always requires temporary pacing post-MI

    e Will usually progress to higher degrees of heart block

Q92 The following drugs will prolong the QT interval:

    a Lithium

    b Terfenadine

    c Quinine

    d Quinidine

    e Amiodarone

Q93 Ventricular fibrillation:

    a Should be treated with an unsynchronised electric shock with an initial energy of 200J; if unsuccessful, a second shock of 200J, and, if necessary, a third shock of 360J

b Should be treated with intra-cardiac calcium injection if DC cardioversion fails after two attempts

c IV amiodarone may be given as 300 mg bolus

d 1 mg IV epinephrine is the drug of choice

e IV atropine sulphate has no role

Q94 Carotid sinus syndrome:

a Is investigated by carotid sinus massage for 5 minutes on each side

b Is common in young adults

c Causes bradycardia as the responsible mechanism for syncope

d Permanent pacemaker insertion is the treatment of choice

e Is a known cause of falls in the elderly without history of syncope

Q95 Ventricular tachycardia:

a Non-sustained VT lasts less than 30 seconds, whereas sustained VT lasts more than 30 seconds

b The vast majority of post-MI VT and VF occur within the first 48 hours of MI

c May be treated with amiodarone 150 mg infused over 10 minutes

d Immediate cardioversion is generally not needed for rates under 150 bpm

e IV beta-blockers have no role

Q96 A 24-year-old student has an ECG with a PR interval of 0.7 s and a QT interval of 0.6 s. Which of the following could be responsible?

a Clopidogrel

b Augmentin

c Erythromycin

d Sotalol

e Digoxin

Q97 A prominent R wave in V1 may occur with which of the following?

a Wolf–Parkinson–White syndrome type A

b RBBB

c Posterior infarction

d Dextrocardia

e Wolf–Parkinson–White syndrome type B

Q98 The most common type of dysrhythmia associated with WPW syndrome is:

a Atrial fibrillation

b Ventricular fibrillation

c Multifocal PVCs

d Atrial tachycardia

e AV-nodal re-entry tachycardia

Q99 Which of the following electrolyte abnormalities may cause long QT segment?

a Hypokalaemia

b Hypocalcaemia

c Hypomagnesaemia

d Hyponatraemia

e Hypernatraemia

Cardiac failure

Q100 Signs of cardiac failure are:

    a   Sinus bradycardia

    b   Increased JVP

    c   Pansystolic murmur

    d   Third heart sound

    e   Fatigue

Q101 Heart failure:

    a   Prevalence is about 1% of the total population

    b   Diagnosis is made clinically and not dependant on the ejection fraction

    c   Has a poor prognosis, with a 5-year mortality of 50%

    d   Treatment with oral frusemide has been shown to decrease mortality by 20%

    e   Beta-blockers are negatively inotropic and should never be used

Q102 Regarding heart failure trials:

    a   CONSENSUS was conducted in 253 patients and demonstrated a reduction in mortality of 31% at 1 year

    b   CONSENSUS used ramipril in patients with severe congestive heart failure (NYHA Class IV)

    c   CONSENSUS II was a large multi-centre trial that also showed a large mortality benefit from early ACE inhibition

    d   Both CONSENSUS & CONSENSUS II were stopped early because of overwhelming benefit in favour of the active drug e Both CONSENSUS & CONSENSUS II were primary prevention heart failure trials

Q103 The SAVE study:

a Was a primary prevention study

b Evaluated captopril starting 3–16 days after MI

c Demonstrated all-cause mortality reduction of 19% in the active drug group

d Showed that the benefit of ACE inhibition in patients with impaired LV dysfunction is confined to those with symptomatic heart failure

e Showed a 24% reduction in the need to undergo revascularisation by PTCA or CABG in the active arm of the trial

Q104 The AIRE study:

a Showed that presence of a single episode of acute pulmonary oedema was enough for entry criteria to the study

b Was a primary prevention study

c Used lisinopril as its active ACE inhibitor

d Showed that the mortality reduction was demonstrated at 6 months post-MI; all patients randomised had confirmed MI by WHO criteria

Endocarditis

Q105 Common signs of endocarditis include:

a Splenomegaly

b Haematuria

c Finger clubbing

d Osler's nodes

e Janeway lesions

Q106 What are features of endocarditis indicating poor prognosis?:

a Negative blood cultures

b Increased PR-Interval on ECG

c Urine output 10 mL/hr

d Splenomegaly

e Finger clubbing

Q107 What are features of endocarditis that warrant surgical intervention?

a First-degree heart block

b Fungal growth on blood cultures

c Pansystolic murmurs

d Fever >38°C for 1 week

e No improvement after 2 weeks IV antibiotics

Q108 In patients with infective endocarditis:

a Cardiac failure is a major cause of death

b Atrial septal defect of secundum type is the most common predisposing congenital lesion c *Staphylococcus aureus* is the most common infecting organism

d Cardiac surgery should not be undertaken until there has been at least two negative blood cultures

e Retinal haemorrhages are a recognised feature

Q109 Endocarditis:

a Can be ruled out if the echocardiogram is normal

b Usually responds to IV antibiotics within 72 hours

c Most abscesses are para-aortic

d Transthoracic echo is superior to transoesphageal echo in diagnosis of vegetations

e Vegetations do not form on a healthy endocardial surface

Interventional cardiology

Q110 Regarding the anatomy of coronary arteries:

    a The circumflex is a branch of the RCA

    b Occlusion of the left main stem results in ST elevation in leads II, III, and AVF

    c LAD runs in the atrio-ventricular groove

    d LAD supplies the LV apex

    e LCx never supplies the AV node

Q111 Coronary stenting:

    a Is associated with lower re-stenosis rate compared with PTCA

    b Patients must be heparinised for 10 days post-stenting

    c In patients prescribed aspirin, they take this for life

    d In patients prescribed clopidogrel, they take this for life

    e In patients prescribed warfarin, they take this for life

Q112 Following PTCA:

    a Patients return to work quicker compared with CABG

    b There is a higher rate of re-stenosis compared with CABG

    c <5% require emergency (females have a higher rate of re-stenosis due to smaller arteries)

    d Patients may drive after 1 week

Q113 What factors are associated with increased risk of post-PTCA restenosis?

    a Diabetes mellitus

    b Continued smoking

c Female sex

d Distal LAD lesion

e Multi-vessel lesion

Q114 Which of the following is the treatment of choice for a 65-year-old patient who has survived an out-of-hospital VF arrest with subsequent normal coronary angiography?

a Amiodarone

b Quinidine

c Procainamide

d Permanent pacemaker

e Implantable cardiac defibrillator

Cardiac surgery

Q115 Complications of CABG include:

a Atrial fibrillation in 25% of cases

b Mediastinitis

c Renal failure

d Phrenic nerve injury

e Psychosis

Q116 Coronary artery bypass surgery has been shown to improve prognosis in patients with:

a 90% stenosis of left main stem

b Triple vessel disease without left main stem isolated RCA lesion

c Ejection fraction less than 30%

d Failed PTCA

Q117 Vessels used as bypass conduits include:

a Left internal mammary artery

b Right internal thoracic artery

c Radial artery

d Superficial femoral artery

e Gastroepiploic artery

Q118 Regarding cardiac surgery:

a Off-pump Coronary Artery Bypass (OPCAB) is associated with fewer complications compared with on-pump CABG

b OPCAB involves stopping the heart using St Thomas' cardioplegia solution

c Pulmonary artery banding for Fallot's tetralogy may be performed through a lateral thoracotomy

d Females have a higher mortality for CABG than males

Q119 Regarding the right dominance of the coronary arterial supply, the posterior interventricular artery is a branch of:

a Left coronary artery

b Right coronary artery

c The circumflex

d Anterior interventricular artery

e Coronary sinus

Q120 Mitral stenosis may present as:

a Tiredness

b Exertional dyspnoea

c Paroxysmal nocturnal dyspnoea

d Haemoptysis

e Right hemipariesis

Q121 Myocarditis:

a May present with a systolic murmur

b Usually causes secondary hypertension

c Causes non-specific ST depression

d Is often caused by Coxsackie virus

e Is worsened by hypoxia

Q122 Clinical features of mitral stenosis include:

a Atrial fibrillation

b Displaced apex beat

c De Musset's sign

d Corrigan's sign

e Ejection systolic murmur with opening snap

Q123 Tetralogy of Fallot is characterised by:

a Atrial septal defects

b Left ventricular hypertrophy

c Pulmonary stenosis

d Patent ductus arteriosus

e Overriding of the pulmonary trunk

Valvular heart disease

Q124 Regarding aortic stenosis:

   a It is typically supravalvular in origin

   b It may be congenital

   c Always requires surgery if gradient is >50 mmHg

   d Is a recognised cause of secondary hypertenison

   e The ECG may be normal

Q125 The Eisenmenger syndrome is pulmonary hypertension with a right to left shunt in association with:

   a Tetralogy of Fallot

   b Patent ductus arteriosus

   c Patent foramen ovale

   d Ventricular septal defect

Q126 Cardiac myxoma:

   a May occur in any cardiac chamber

   b 85% occur in the right atrium

   c May recur after surgical resection

   d Cardiac catheterization data is usually always required

   e May cause an opening snap on auscultation

Q127 Artificial heart valves:

a Xenografts do not need warfarin anticoagulation

b Xenografts deteriorate faster in younger patients

c Xenografts deteriorate faster during pregnancy

d A re-do mitral valve replacement carries twice the risk of a re-do aortic valve replacement

e Warfarin crosses the placenta

Q128 Hypertension in pregnancy:

a Beta-blockers are contraindicated

b ACE inhibitors are contraindicated

c Methyldopa is safe and effective

d Diazepam is the first-line agent for eclampsia

Q129 Transposition of the Great Arteries (TGA):

a Is more common in females

b Occurs in 1 in 4500 live births

c Birth weight is usually normal

d Presents at birth

e If present without a shunt, may present in early adulthood

Q130 Ventricular septal defect:

a Is the most common cyanotic congenital heart lesion

b Occurs in 2 per 1000 live births

c Is the most common muscular type of defect

d Spontaneous closure occurs in 30–50% of cases

e 50% of spontaneous closure occurs in the first year of life

Q131 The drug of choice for a 30-week pregnant woman with essential hypertension and no signs of eclampsia is:

  a Propranolol

  b Amlodipine

  c Methyldopa

  d Ramipril

  e Valsartan

Q132 The following changes occur during pregnancy:

  a Cardiac output decreases

  b Apex beat displaces laterally

  c Persistent sinus tachycardia develops

  d Cardiomegaly develops

  e Systolic BP decreases during the second trimester

Q133 Features of Tetralogy of Fallot are:

  a Ventricular septal defect

  b Atrial septal defect

  c Right ventricular hypertrophy

  d Aortic stenosis

  e Patent foramen ovale

Cardiorespiratory physiology

Q134 In a standard 70 kg male:

a Approximately 60% of body weight is water

b Sodium is the predominant extracellular ion

c Most of the calcium ions in the body are located intracellularly

d Normal intracranial pressure is 10 mmHg

e 75% of the total body water is extracellular

Q135 During the cardiac cycle, the maximal right ventricular systolic pressure is:

a 4 mmHg

b 10 mmHg

c 25 mmHg

d 60 mmHg

e 120 mmHg

Q136 The QRS complex:

a Has a normal duration of 0.3 s

b Represents ventricular depolarisation

c Represents ventricular systole

d Represents atrial relaxation

e Represents atrial repolarisation

Q137 The Cardiac index:

a Increases within age

b Is synonymous with cardiac output

c Is cardiac output divided by body mass index

d Is cardiac output per square metre of body surface area

e Is stroke volume times heart rate

Q138 Regarding the neuromuscular junction:

a Dopamine is the principal neurotransmitter

b Dopamine is an inhibitory neurotransmitter

c Dopamine is converted into adrenaline

d A suxamethonium molecule is two acetylcholine molecules joined together

e Transmission is inhibited by calcium ions

Q139 Which of the following conditions does *not* induce cor pulmonale?

a Bronchial asthma

b Left atrial myxoma

c Pickwickian syndrome

d Fibrosing alveolitis

e Syphilitic aortitis

Q140 The oxyhaemoglobin dissociation curve is shifted to the left by:

a A fall in pH

b Foetal haemoglobin

c Increased body temperature

d Increased PCO_2

e Increased 2,3-diphosphoglycerate

Q141 Starling's law of the heart:

   a Is not applicable during exercise

   b Explains the increase in heart rate during exercise

   c Explains the increase in cardiac output when venous return increases

   d Explains the increase in cardiac output due to sympathetic stimulation

   e Is not obeyed by the failing heart

Q142 In the left lateral position, blood flow to the non-dominant lung is?

   a 25%

   b 35%

   c 45%

   d 55%

   e 65%

Q143 Pulmonary surfactant:

   a Is produced by type II pneumocytes

   b Is produced so rapidly that a decreased blood flow can decrease production

   c Synthesis is stimulated by thyroxine

   d Is metabolised by endocytosis

Q144 Acidosis may result in:

   a Hyperkalaemia

   b Increased chloride ions

c Decreased PCO_2

d Tetany

Q145 The cardiovascular response to cooling a healthy patient to 32°C is?

a Bradycardia

b Prolongation of the PR-interval

c Prolongation of the QT-interval

d Ventricular fibrillation

Q146 Which of the following is a risk factor for increased susceptibility for drug-induced torsades de pointes?

a Being female

b Hypokalaemia

c Hypomagnesaemia

d Sinus tachycardia

Q147 In adults, the angle at which the right main bronchus leaves the carina is?

a 15 degrees

b 20 degrees

c 25 degrees

d 30 degrees

Q148 Myocardial contractility is increased by?

    a Tachycardia

    b Catecholamines

    c Increased vagal activity

    d Increased cardiac muscle fibre length

    e Increased calcium ions

Q149 Sinus arrhythmia:

    a Is more common in the elderly

    b Increases the R-R interval

    c Is maximal with breath holding

    d Is more common during exercise

    e Causes QT prolongation

Q150 Which of the following are precursors of adrenaline?

    a Tyrosine

    b Phenylalanine

    c Noradrenaline

    d Dopamine

    e Isoprenaline

Explanatory answers

Cardiac glycosides

A1 a False Digoxin *increases* the PR interval.

   b True

   c True Digoxin, especially at toxicity levels, may cause any cardiac arrhythmia, including atrial fibrillation.

   d True

   e False

A2 a True

   b True

   c True

   d True

   e True

A3 a False Digoxin is a cardiac glycoside that acts by inhibiting Na/K-ATPase. H/K-ATPase is the proton pump, inhibited by proton pump inhibitors such as omperazole.

   b False

   c False

   d True

   e False Digoxin serum concentrations peak within 1–3 hours.

A4 a False The results of the Digitalis Intervention Group (DIG) Trial showed that digoxin reduced the number of hospital admissions but did *not* reduce mortality.

   b False Both digoxin and verapamil are specifically contraindicated in WPW syndrome.

   c True RELIANCE study.

   d False May result in hypokalaemia.

   e False

A5 a True

      b False

      c True   Verapamil can reduce the renal excretion of digoxin by up to 100%.

      d False There is no specific interaction here.

      e True   Dehydration secondary to acute infection may precipitate digoxin toxicity.

A6 a True

      b True

      c True

      d True

      e True

A7 a True

      b True

      c True

      d False

A8 a False

      b False

      c False

      d True

Diuretics

A9 a False Frusemide is a *loop* diuretic.

      b False

      c True

      d False Loop diuretics act by inhibiting *active* sodium reabsorption in the *thick* segment of the *ascending* Loop of Henle.

      e True

A10 a False Hyperglycaemia.

      b True

      c True

      d False Hypercalcaemia.

      e False May precipitate gout.

A11 a False

      b False

      c False

      d True

      e False

A12 a False

      b False

      c False

      d False

      e False

A13 a False

b False

c False

d False

e False

A14 a False

b True

c False

d True

e False

Beta-adrenoceptor blocking drugs

A15　a　True

　　　b　False

　　　c　False

　　　d　False

　　　e　True　The absolute contraindication.

A16　a　True

　　　b　False　Beta-blockers may mask the warning signs of hypoglycaemia but are *not* specifically contraindicated in diabetic patients.

　　　c　False　Despite popular belief, there is *no* specific evidence to support this.

　　　d　False　No specific evidence here.

　　　e　False

A17　a　False

　　　b　True

　　　c　True

　　　d　False

　　　e　False

A18　a　False　There is no clinical trial demonstrating statistically significant mortality reductions with atenolol.

　　　b　True　BHAT study showed positive outcome.

　　　c　True

　　　d　True　The recently published CAPRICORN study demonstrated all-cause mortality reduction with statistical significance with carvedilol.

　　　e　False　MIAMI trial demonstrated benefit but was not statistically significant.

A19 a True   Propranolol is a lipid-soluble drug.

        b False Propranolol is a short-acting drug.

        c False Propranolol may cause lethargy and bradycardia but is *not* a recognised cause of hypothyroidism.

        d True

        e True

A20 a True

        b True

        c True

        d True

        e False

A21 a True

        b True

        c True

        d False

        e False

Calcium-channel antagonists

A22 a False Constipation is most common.

    b False

    c False May precipitate digoxin toxicity.

    d False

    e True

A23 a True

    b False

    c True

    d False

    e False Common with nitrates.

A24 a False

    b False

    c True

    d True

    e False

A25 a True

    b False 35–50 hours.

    c False Starting dose 5 mg daily.

    d False

    e True See PRAISE trial.

A26 a False

b True

c False

d True

e False Mainly liver metabolism.

A27 a True

b True

c False Half-life 1 hour.

d False

e False

A28 a False

b True Cimetidine. By cP450 induction.

c False

d False

e False

ACE inhibitors

A29 a True

b True

c True

d False

e False

A30 a True   Cough occurs in approximately 10% of cases.

b False   Cause hyperkalaemia.

c True

d False

e False

A31 a False   Trandolapril.

b True

c True

d False

e False

A32 a True

b True

c True

d True

e False   1.2% developed cough.

A33 a False

b False

c False

d True

e False

A34 a False   All such patients were excluded.

b True

c True

d True

e True

Statins

A35 a True

　　b False　Simvastatin is a specific inhibitor of HMG-CoA reductase, the enzyme that catalyzes the conversion of HMG-CoA to mevalonate. This process occurs in the liver.

　　c False　The maximum therapeutic response occurs in about 4–6 weeks.

　　d False　Atherosclerosis is a chronic process and the discontinuation of lipid-lowering drugs during pregnancy will have little impact on the outcome of long-term therapy of primary hypercholesterolaemia. Moreover, cholesterol and other products of the cholesterol biosynthesis pathway are essential components for foetal development, including synthesis of steroids and cell membranes. Due to the ability of statins to inhibit this process, it is possible that this may cause harm when administered to a pregnant woman. Therefore, statins are contraindicated during pregnancy and in nursing mothers.

　　e False　May occur in about 1 in 100 000 patient-years.

A36 a True　10 mg atorvastatin produces the most dramatic reduction.

　　b True

　　c True　Similarly neither does cerivastatin.

　　d True

A37 a False　Patients were not post-MI.

　　b False　Pravastatin.

　　c False

　　d True

　　e True

A38 a False Secondary prevention trial.

    b False Simvastatin versus placebo.

    c True

    d True

    e False Extremely rare (1 in 100 000).

A39 a True

    b True

    c False Cholesterol levels 4.0–7.0 mmol/L.

    d False Decreased overall mortality by 22%.

    e False MI or unstable angina.

Thrombolytics

A40 a False

      b True

      c False

      d False

      e False

A41 a True

      b True

      c True

      d False

      e False

A42 a True

      b True

      c False

      d True

      e True   As TPA has the shortest half-life.

A43 a True

      b True

      c True

      d True   Re-perfusion arrhythmia.

      e True

A44 a False Anistreplase was used.

b True

c True

d False Heparin not part of protocol.

e True

A45 a True

b False

c True

d True

e False

Anti-platelet agents

A46 a True

b False

c False Cyclo-oxygenase inhibitor.

d False May have benefit at 3 mg daily.

e False

A47 a True

b False TARGET study showed Reopro better.

c False

d False

e False

A48 a True

b True

c True

d False No significant differences.

e False This is abciximab.

Inotropes

A49 a False   Renal dose is 'low' dose (1–5 mcg/kg/min).

      b False

      c False   Must be given via central line.

      d False

      e True

A50 a True

      b True

      c True   Good second-line agent for bradycardia.

      d True

      e True

A51 a True   Also called 'deadly nightshade'.

      b True

      c True

      d True

      e False   Causes pupil dilation.

A52 a True

      b True

      c False

      d False

      e True

A53 a True

      b True

      c True

d False

e True

A54 a False

b True

c False

d False

e False

A55 a True

b False

c True

d False

e True

A56 a True

b False

c True

d False

e True

Anti-dysrythmic drugs

A57 a True

      b True

      c True

      d True

      e True

A58 a False

      b False

      c False

      d True

      e True

A59 a True

      b True

      c True

A60 a True

      b True

      c True

      d False

      e True

A61 a True

      b False

      c False

      d True

      e False

A62 a False

b False

c False

d False It occurs but is not common!

e True

A63 a True

b True

c True

d False

e False

A64 a True

b True

c True

d False Occurs with *hyperkalaemia*.

e False

A65 a True

b True

c True

d True

e True

A66 a False

b False

c True

d True

e True

Acute myocardial infarction

A67 a True

  b False A number of studies have demonstrated in-hospital mortality of about 20%.

  c True Especially with diabetic patients.

  d True Rare presentation but well documented.

  e True

A68 a True

  b True

  c True

  d True

  e True

A69 a False

  b False The prognosis for an individual patient can be accurately estimated simply by the ST segment deviation present in one ECG lead recorded 90 minutes after thrombolysis.

  c False

  d False

  e False

A70 a False

  b True

  c False

  d False

  e False

A71 a False The first dose of captopril was rapidly titrated to 50 mg bd with the first dose given within 2 hours of thrombolysis.

 b False There was no evidence of benefit from mortality reduction using IV nitrates.

 c True

 d True

 e False

A72 a False

 b True

 c False

 d False

 e False

A73 a True

 b False

 c False

 d False

 e False

A74 a True

 b True

 c False

 d False

 e False

Hypertension

A75 a True Essential hypertension.

b True

c False

d False 20% of population.

e False Tends to cause hypokalaemia.

A76 a True

b False

c False

d False

e False

A77 a False

b False

c False

d True

A78 a True

b True 10% of cases.

c True

d False May cause hyperkalaemia.

e True

A79 a True

b True

c True

d False SHEP trial.

e False

A80 a False

a True

b False

c False

d False

A81 a True

b True

c False

d True

e True

A82 a False   Beta-blockers are contraindicated in asthma.

b False   May precipitate gout.

c False

d True

e False

A83 a False

b True

c False

d False

e False

A84 a False

b False

c False

d False

e True   Drug-induced SLE is likely here.

Atrial fibrillation

A85 a False AF may complicate acute MI infarction in 10–15%
of cases and is often a marker of extensive myocardial
damage and of poor prognosis with associated
increased mortality.

    b True

    c True

    d False

    e True

A86 a True

    b True

    c True Especially paroxysmal AF.

    d True

    e True

A87 a True

    b True

    c True Approximately 30–40% of its structure.

    d False

    e True

A88 a False

    b True

    c False

    d True

    e False Caused by vancomycin.

A89 a True

b True

c False   Target 2.0–2.5 INR.

d True

e False

Dysrhythmias

A90 a True

b False

c True

d True

e True

A91 a False   Right coronary artery (RCA).

b True   Due to occluded RCA.

c False

d False

e False

A92 a True

b True   Now discontinued.

c True   Used for nocturnal cramps.

d True

e True

A93 a True

b False

c False   Not beneficial.

d True   No longer called adrenaline.

e True

A94 a True

b True

c False

d True

e False

A95 a False

b False

c False

d False

e True

A96 a False

b False

c True

d False

e False

A97 a False

b True

c True

d True

e True

A98 a False

b False

c False

d False

e True

A99 a True

    b True

    c True

    d False

    e False

Cardiac failure

A100 a False Sinus tachycardia.

     b True

     c False Indicates other cardiac pathology.

     d True

     e True

A101 a True

     b True

     c True

     d False No mortality benefit.

     e False Only to be specifically avoided in overt heart failure.

A102 a True

     b False Enalapril (consENsus).

     c False

     d False Only CONSENSUS was terminated early.

     e False

A103 a False

     b True

     c True

     d False Benefit also conferred to asymptomatic patients.

     e True

A104 a True

b False

c False   Ramipril.

d False

Endocarditis

A105 a True

  b True

  c False Only 10% have finger clubbing.

  d False Very rare sign.

  e False Very rare sign.

A106 a True

  b True

  c True

  d False

  e False

A107 a True

  b True

  c False

  d False

  e False

A108 a True

  b False

  c False *Streptococcus viridans.*

  d False

  e True

A109 a False

b True

c True

d False

e False Less commonly.

Interventional cardiology

A110 a False

   b False ST elevation in II, III, AVF implies RCA territory infarct.

   c False Interventricular groove.

   d True

   e False AV nodal branch of RCA.

A111 a False 0.1%.

   b False 0.1–0.2%.

   c False 0.1%.

   d True

   e False

A112 a True

   b False

   c True

   d False

A113 a True

   b True

   c True

   d False

   e False

A114 a False
b False
c False
d False
e True

Cardiac surgery

A115 a True

b True

c True

d True

e True

A116 a True

b True

c False

d False

A117 a True

b True

c True

d False

e True

A118 a True

b False

c True

d True

A119 a False

b True

c False

d False

e False

A120 a True

b False

c False

d True

e True

A121 a True

b False

c True

d True

e True

A122 a True Due to enlarged L atrium.

b False Mitral stenosis causes a non-displaced tapping apex beat.

c False May indicate aortic regurgitation.

d False Corrigan's sign of visible neck pulsation is a sign of aortic regurgitation.

e False The murmur of mitral stenosis is typically mid-diastolic.

A123 a False

b False

c True

d False

e False

Valvular heart disease

A124 a False

    b True

    c False

    d False

    e True

A125 a False

    b False

    c False

    d True VSD is part of Eisenmenger's complex.

A126 a True

    b False 85% in left atrium.

    c True

    d False

    e False Suggests mitral stenosis.

A127 a True

    b True

    c True

    d True

    e True

A128 a False

    b True Known teratogen.

    c True

    d False

A129 a False More common in males.

b True

c True

d True

e False Not compatible with life.

A130 a False Most common congential lesion.

b True

c False

d True

e True

A131 a False

b False

c True

d False

e False

A132 a False Increases.

b True Laterally and upwards.

c False

d True

e True

A133 a True

b False

c True

d False

e False

Cardiorespiratory physiology

A134 a True

      b True

      c False

      d True

      e False

A135 a False

      b False

      c True

      d False

      e False

A136 a False

      b True

      c False

      d False

      e False

A137 a False

      b False

      c False

      d True

      e False

A138 a False

b True

c True

d True

e False

A139 a False

b False

c False

d False

e True

A140 a False

b True

c False

d False

e False

A141 a False

b False

c True

d False

e False

A142 a True

b False

c False

d False

e False

A143 a True

      b True

      c True

      d True

A144 a True

      b True

      c True

      d False

A145 a True

      b True

      c True

      d False

A146 a True

      b True

      c True

      d True

A147 a False

      b False

      c True

      d False

A148 a True

b True

c True

d False

e True

A149 a False

b True

c False

d False

e False

A150 a True

b True

c True

d True

e False

References

Q1

Campbell RW. Whither digitalis? *Lancet*. 1997; **349**: 1854–5.

Q4

Garg R, Gorlin R, Smith T, *et al.*, for the Digitalis Investigation Group. The effect of digoxin on mortality and morbidity in patients with heart failure. *N Engl J Med*. 1997; **336**: 525–33.

Packer M, Gheorghiade M, Young JB, *et al.* Withdrawal of digoxin from patients with chronic heart failure treated with angiotensin-converting-enzyme inhibitors. RADIANCE Study. *N Engl J Med*. 1993; **329**: 1–7.

Q18

Freemantle N, *et al.* Blockade after myocardial infarction: systematic review and meta regression analysis. *BMJ*. 1999; **318**: 1730–7.

Anon. Timolol-induced reduction in mortality and reinfarction in patients surviving acute myocardial infarction. *N Engl J Med*. 1981; **304**: 801–7.

Hjalmarson A, Elmfeldt D, Herlitz J, *et al.* Effect on mortality of metoprolol in acute myocardial infarction: a double-blind randomised trial. *Lancet*. 1981; **2**: 823–7.

Pedersen TR. Six-year follow-up of the Norwegian Multicenter Study on Timolol after acute myocardial infarction. *N Engl J Med*. 1985; **313**: 1055–8.

Beta-blocker Heart Attack Study Group. The beta-blocker heart attack trial. *JAMA*. 1981; **246**: 2073–4.

Q20

GREAT Group. Feasibility, safety, and efficacy of domiciliary thrombolysis by general practitioners: Grampian Region Early Anistreplase Trial. *BMJ*. 1992; **305**: 548–53.

The MIAMI Trial Research Group. Metoprolol in acute myocardial infarction: patient population. *Am J Cardiol*. 1985; **56**: 1G–57G.

Anon. ISIS-4: a randomised factorial trial assessing early oral captopril, oral mononitrate, and intravenous magnesium sulphate in 58,050 patients with suspected acute myocardial infarction. *Lancet*. 1995; **345**: 669–85.

Q21

Cleland JG, Swedberg K. Carvedilol for heart failure, with care. *Lancet*. 1996; **347**: 1199–201.

Q22

Kelly JG, O'Malley K. Clinical pharmacokinetics of calcium antagonists: an update. *Clin Pharmacokinet*. 1992; **22**: 416–21.

Q23

Dollery CT. Clinical pharmacology of the calcium antagonists. *Am J Hypertens*. 1991; **4**: 88S–95S.

Q24

Gibson RS, Boden WE, Theroux P, *et al*. Diltiazem and reinfarction in patients with non-Q-wave myocardial infarction: results of a double-blind, randomised, multicenter trial. *N Engl J Med.* 1986; **315**: 423–9.

Q32

Ambrosioni E, Borghi C, Magnani B. The effect of the angiotensin-converting-enzyme inhibitor zofenopril on mortality and morbidity after anterior myocardial infarction: the Survival of Myocardial Infarction: Long-Term Evaluation (SMILE) Study Investigators. *N Engl J Med.* 1995; **332**: 80–5.

Q34

The Heart Outcomes Prevention Evaluation (HOPE) study investigators. *N Engl J Med.* 2000; **342**: 145–53.

Q35

Simvastatin (Zocor) Data sheet. Merck, Sharp & Dohme (MSD); 1991.

Q37

Sacks FM, Pfeffer MA, Braunwald E, *et al.*, for the CARE Investigators. *Effect of pravastatin on coronary events after myocardial infarction in patients with average cholesterol levels: preliminary results of the Cholesterol and Recurrent Events (CARE) trial.* Presented at the American College of Cardiology Annual Scientific Session; March 1996.

Q38

Anon. Randomised trial of cholesterol lowering in 4444 patients with coronary heart disease: the Scandinavian Simvastatin Survival Study (4S). *Lancet*. 1994; **344**: 1383–9.

Q39

The Long-Term Intervention with Pravastatin in Ischaemic Disease (LIPID) Study Group. Prevention of cardiovascular events and death with pravastatin in patients with coronary heart disease and a broad range of initial cholesterol levels. *N Engl J Med*. 1998; **339**: 1349–57.

Cannon CP, Weintraub WS, Demopoulos LA, *et al*. Invasive versus conservative strategies in unstable angina and non-Q wave myocardial infarction following treatment with tirofiban: rationale and study design of the international TACTICS-TIMI 18 Trial: Treat Angina with Aggrastat and determine Cost of Therapy with an Invasive or Conservative Strategy: Thrombolysis in Myocardial Infarction. *Am J Cardiol*. 1998; **82**: 731–6.

Q42

Barr P, Berry A. *Drug Therapy in Newborn Infants: prescribing information*. Sydney: Royal Alexandra Hospital for Children; 1994.

Q45

Warkentin TE, Levine MN, Hirsh J, *et al*. Heparin-induced thrombocytopenia in patients treated with low-molecular-weight heparin or unfractionated heparin. *N Engl J Med*. 1995; **332**: 1330–5.

Q46

Anon. Ticlopidine versus aspirin for the prevention of recurrent stroke: analysis of patients with minor stroke from the Ticlopidine Aspirin Stroke Study. *Stroke*. 1992; **23**(12): 1723–7.

Anon. The Canadian American Ticlopidine Study (CATS) in thromboembolic stroke. *Lancet*. 1989; **1**: 1215–20.

Q48

PURSUIT Trial Investigators. Inhibition of platelet glycoprotein IIb/IIIa with eptifibatide in patients with acute coronary syndromes. Platelet glycoprotein IIb/IIIa in unstable angina: receptor suppression using integrilin therapy. *N Engl J Med*. 1998; **339**: 436–43.

Q51

Gunnar RM, Bourdillon PDV, Dixon DW, *et al*. Guidelines for the early management of patients with acute myocardial infarction: a report of the American College of Cardiology/American Heart Association Task Force on Assessment of Diagnostic and Therapeutic Cardiovascular Procedures (Subcommittee to Develop Guidelines for the Early Management of Patients with Acute Myocardial Infarction). *J Am Coll Cardiol*. 1990; **16**: 249–52.

Q54

Anon. ISIS-4: a randomised factorial trial assessing early oral captopril, oral mononitrate, and intravenous magnesium sulphate in 58,050 patients with suspected acute myocardial infarction. *Lancet*. 1995; **345**: 669–85.

Q55

Al-Mohammed A. Prevalence of hibernating myocardium in patients with severely impaired ischaemic left ventricles. *Heart*. 1998; **80**: 559–64.

Q61

Schröder K, Wegscheider K, Zeymer U, *et al*. Extent of ST-segment deviation in a single electrocardiogram lead 90 min after thrombolysis as a predictor of medium-term mortality in acute myocardial infarction. *Lancet*. 2001; **358**: 1479–86.

Epstein AE, Hallstrom AP, Rogers WJ, *et al*. Mortality following ventricular arrhythmia suppression by encainide, flecainide, and moricizine after myocardial infarction: the original design concept of the Cardiac Arrhythmia Suppression Trial (CAST). *JAMA*. 1993; **270**: 2451–5.

Sugiura T, Iwasaka T, Takahashi N, *et al*. Atrial fibrillation in inferior wall Q-wave acute myocardial infarction. *Am J Cardiol*. 1991; **67**: 1135–6.

Q65

Behar S, Tanne D, Zion M, *et al*. Incidence and prognostic significance of chronic atrial fibrillation among 5839 consecutive patients with acute myocardial infarction: the SPRINT Study Group. Secondary Prevention Reinfarction Israeli Nifedipine Trial. *Am J Cardiol*. 1992; **70**: 816–18.

Q69

American Heart Association, Emergency Cardiac Care Committee and Subcommittees. Guidelines for cardiopulmonary resuscitation and emergency cardiac care, part III: adult advanced cardiac life support. *JAMA*. 1992; **268**: 2199–241.

Q70

Campbell RW, Murray A, Julian DG. Ventricular arrhythmias in first 12 hours of acute myocardial infarction: natural history study. *Br Heart J*. 1981; **46**: 351–7.

Nademanee K, Taylor RD, Bailey WM. Management and long-term outcome of patients with electrical storm. *J Am Coll Cardiol*. 1995; **25**: 187A.

Q102

Sigurdsson A, Swedberg K. Left ventricular remodelling, neurohormonal activation and early treatment with enalapril (CONSENSUS II) following myocardial infarction. *Eur Heart J*. 1994; **15**(suppl B): 14–19.

Q103

Pfeffer MA, Braunwald E, Moye LA, *et al*. Effect of captopril on mortality and morbidity in patients with left ventricular dysfunction after myocardial infarction: results of the survival and ventricular enlargement trial – the SAVE Investigators. *N Engl J Med*. 1992; **327**: 669–77.

Q104

The Acute Infarction Ramipril Efficacy (AIRE) Study Investigators. Effect of ramipril on mortality and morbidity of survivors of acute myocardial infarction with clinical evidence of heart failure. *Lancet*. 1993; **342**: 821–8.

Q109

Oakley CM, Hall RJC. Endocarditis: problem-patients being treated for endocarditis and not doing well. *Heart*. 2001; **85**: 470–4.

Q110

Baroldi G. Disease of the coronary arteries. In: Silver MD, editor. *Cardiovascular Pathology, Vol 1*. New York: Churchill Livingstone; 1983. pp. 317–91.

Index